AskDoctorPam
About Mental Health

Pamula Mills, Ph.D.

All Rights Reserved. No part of this book may be reproduced or transmitted in any form or any manner, electronic of mechanical, including photocopying, recording or by any information storage and retrieval system, without permission in writing from the author and/or publisher.

Published by:
Ellis & Ellis Consulting Group, LLC
954-439-0760

Copyright © 2023. Pamula Mills, Ph.D.

ISBN 13- 9798379394707

10- 9798379394

Printed in the United States of America.

Acknowledgements

This book is dedicated to the memory of my parents, Bishop Sammy, and Lady Irene Ellis, my siblings, Jackson, Boldrage, Dinnie, Rumalo and Bercu, and to all of my surviving siblings.

Forever my girls-Damali, Dhara and Jani and our pet Chihuahua, Teddy Bear.

Thank you, Chay, Cecil Thompson, Damaris Thompson, R.H., A.R., R.M., my friends, supporters, encouragers, prayer partners and readership.

Truth

If one mans says it, it is your word against his.
If a second man says it, whose word is?
If a third man says it, it's time to be true;
The one denying is probably you.
Dr. Pam

Taking care of one's mental health, speaks truth to power.
Living the most authentic life requires a balance of body, mind, and spirit.

Introduction

In 2000, Dr. Pam returned to her island nation, The Bahamas, after pursuing a terminal degree in Clinical Psychology and Family Therapy, in the United States. She settled in Freeport, Grand Bahama, where she assumed the role of Supervisor of Special Services, in the Ministry of Education. This position also included providing services to the islands of Abaco and Bimini, Bahamas. She was responsible for School Psychological Services, School Guidance and Counseling Services, School Attendance, Special Education and Employee Assistance Services.

Dr. Pam remained in Grand Bahama until 2016. During her tenure in the Bahamas, she graciously offered her services to the community. In addition to being an adjunct professor at the College (now university) of The

Bahamas, Dr. Pam is the founder of the island's crisis team, P.A.R.T. (Professional Assistance and Restoration Team, 2001), a community-based organization that was established to assist with many of the island's critical situations. In 2019, following the passage of Hurricane Dorian, she returned to Grand Bahama to rejuvenate the crisis team, which continues to function today, in part.

While in Grand Bahama, Dr. Pam had the opportunity to conduct numerous conferences, workshops, and training, in all areas of mental health. This culminated in a weekly radio show, with her colleague, Mrs. Joyce Pinder, following the passage of Hurricanes Jeanne, Francis, and Wilma, in 2004 and 2005, called, "Helping, Healing and Restoration." This radio show was well received by the community and ran for several years. During this time, Dr. Pam did many television and public appearances, schools, civic organizations, and church presentations, speaking engagements and consultations, educating people on the importance of taking care of their mental health.

Being very concerned about the 'stigma' attached to mental health Dr. Pam had an idea. She wanted to give information on mental health, 'without throwing it in people's faces,' or overwhelming them. In 2006, she approached the editors of The Freeport News about writing a weekly column with nuggets and information on mental health, that would be identifiable and appreciated by all; hence, AskDoctorPam was born as a special column, presented on Tuesdays, and continued until 2019, when The Freeport News was destroyed by Hurricane Dorian. The column was fueled in two ways; letters were written to and answered by Dr. Pam, and Dr. Pam wrote nuggets of information to the public, hidden in cultural, personal, professional, or societal stories, often with a humorous twist, but always with pertinent, relevant information. Each article featured a "Point to Ponder," which was a catchy phrase, that summarized the content of the article, and gave the reader something to take away.

Today, Dr. Pam presents a collection of these articles. Which have been categorized under several topics, AskDoctorPam about anything. In addition to "Points to Ponder", there is a blank page called, "Notes of Reflection," after each article, for the reader to record personal thoughts, take aways and impressions. Questions or inquiries for Dr. Pam may be emailed to *askdoctorpam@yahoo.com*.

AskDoctorPam – About Mental Health

It's Just a Matter of Time

Dear Readers,

We recently observed another anniversary of the death of Marvin Gaye. Gaye, was an African American Rhythm and Blues singer of the 60's and 70's, who became very popular with such hits as "Heard it Through the Grapevine, Sexual Healing, What's Going On and Lets Get it On." He had a sultry, distinguishable voice that left its listeners feeling special and mellow.

What was significant about Gaye's death, was the way he died. He was shot by his father, while attempting to intervene in an argument between his parents. His father contended that the death was an accident; he, however (father), served time in jail for the shooting and died some years upon release. This incident divided the Gaye family and left many wondering how such a tragedy could occur.

Truthfully, we have known of several cases of relatives turning on each other and have seen the added grief and sorrow such actions have rendered on surviving family members. No one wins in these situations. A common explanation is usually not readily found, as each case is different. There are, however, some trends to which we can pay attention.

Firstly, let us establish the fact that every family has issues, and each handles things in its unique way. Pay attention to how your family resolves issues. You will never all agree with any particular point, so sometimes simple things can escalate into arguments. Doing such times, it is a good idea to listen to each other. If this is difficult to do, then ask for a time out from the situation, to revisit when calmer heads prevail. If this is not accomplishable, take responsibility and excuse yourself.

Secondly, know the person with whom you are having heated exchanges. If the other individual is one who gets angry easily, or has a temper or anger problem, be careful about picking physical arguments. Instead, you may want to leave a clear note about your issue or concern, identifying a later time for which to have the discussion. This gives everyone an opportunity to make mental preparations for his/her case.

Thirdly, know yourself and how you resolve conflicts. If you get hot headed, or are often unreasonable, take some time to deal with self. Be honest with self. Talk to someone about your emotions when dealing with others and get some help. Practice staying calm and learn breathing and other soothing techniques.

Fourthly, it is wise to note where you have a discussion that can escalate. If you know the other person, (or you), is prone to throwing items when you speak, a place like the living room where there are many loose items (figurines, vases, etc.), may not be a wise venue. By the same token, the kitchen area where heavier and more dangerous items are kept, may not be the best place either.

Fifthly, always have a quick path for escape. Having a heated argument in a bedroom or bathroom where there is no exit door, leaves you or the person with whom you are arguing, in an extremely vulnerable state. The chances for outside help are less, especially if the door to the room has been closed.

Finally, know patterns. Anyone who makes threats, will soon deliver on these threats. Moreover, anyone who hits, punches, slaps, flashes knives, sharp objects, or a gun, is a deadly person. Do not remain in that relationship; **IT'S JUST A MATTER OF TIME!**

The bottom line is that anyone can cross the line from 'normal' behaviors, or simply SNAP. If you, however, live around a situation that has a history of escalation, pay attention to the patterns, watch your actions and make a plan of escape. Listen to the words that are being said, "I will choke, slap, or kill you," and take these words seriously. Take care of yourself and use wisdom. It is better to be wrong and alive, than right and dead.

Most importantly, cleanse your soul and heart of negative thoughts, deeds and actions that may fester and harbor and bring about unproductive endings. See things for what they truly are presenting.

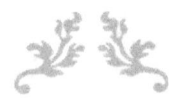

POINT TO PONDER:

Staying aware may help

you stay alive.

Notes of Reflection

AskDoctorPam – About Mental Health

A Dark Hole

Dear Readers,

I watched an episode of the "Mann's" which dealt with 'conquering fears.' David Mann, who confessed to having a fear of enclosed places, was locked in a casket that was measured for his size and weight; there was no room for error. Two small holes were drilled into the top of the box to accommodate breathing. He had to remain in this dark place for one minute. It was difficult and he was three quarters of the way there, when his son, David Junior, decided to place a white mouse, another of David Senior's fears, into the box, through one of the breathing holes. Suffice it to say, the competition was now over; that dark place became a nightmare.

One day, upon completing personal devotions, I was led to telephone a friend, whom I had not seen in several months and who lived abroad. After a brief chit chat of 'catch ups and niceties," she confessed that she was delighted to hear from me and proceeded to tell me about the last few months of her life.

She described her life as being in a dark hole with very few, if any, images about forward mobility. She talked about not wanting to talk to anyone, not answering her phone, canceling dates with friends, little desire to go to work or church, avoiding her friends, staying in bed all day, feeling down and moody, refusing to open windows to allow light to flow into the house and declaring that her life seemed hopeless. I gently informed her, that we often refer to this as DEPRESSION.

She took a long pause and then continued by saying that she decided that she needed to see a professional and had made an appointment to do just that. I was relieved by the last disclosure and encouraged her to do the same. Her decision to seek professional help was strengthened when she realized that I did not judge her, leading her to acknowledge that this was the reason she avoided her friends. We spoke for several minutes more, I prayed with her, she thanked me for calling and we hung up.

I realized that my friend was extremely depressed and cherished the few minutes we shared. More importantly, her resistance to reach out to local friends for the fear of being judged or ridiculed, was a sad reality. This was particularly concerning for her, as she is a Christian follower and felt that fellow Christians would have clichéd her to death (no pun intended), with spiritual quotes. This thought left me perplexed.

Being depressed can feel like being in a dark hole. It can render emotions of hopelessness, despair, desperation loneliness and fear; it is real. Additionally, ANYONE can feel depressed, or extremely sad. It is vital, therefore to know the signs and become aware. Paying attention to life's patterns and making good choices, can keep you ahead of the game. Also, knowing your strengths, limitations and vulnerabilities can prove to be useful.

Depression can happen at any time, but is usually preceded by some traumatic or eventful occasion in one's life. Sometimes it is difficult to explain these feelings to others and the behaviors that follow can seem strange or foreign. Lack of concern, understanding and support, can exacerbate the case, leaving the victim susceptible to undesirable thoughts and actions.

Strive to be as knowledgeable of depression and take care of self. Be that individual who reaches out to others; just as importantly, be that non-judgmental person whom others can reach out and touch.

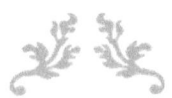

POINT TO PONDER: A dark hole can be a scary place.

Notes of Reflection

Embracing Changes

Dear Readers,

In today's world, change has become the status quo. To survive, both professionally and emotionally, you have to learn how to respond when change happens to you.

Confusion, depression, and fear often accompany change. Whether it's change at work or home, people often feel alone in their situation. The fact is, we all experience similar feelings when coping with difficult changes.

Whenever life acts we respond. If you win the lottery you might be happy. If you lose your job you might become angry. Whatever your reaction, depends upon your attitude. Fortunately, we control our attitudes.

In determining how we face life, it is our attitude that is the key determinant. See whether or not you agree with the following statement.

"You are responsible for all of your experiences of life."

Change is particularly prevalent at middle adult hood, and is noticeable in the physical, cognitive, personality, spiritual and social arenas. This period generally coincides with retirement from a career or vocation that may have dominated a person's life for a significant period of time.

Retiring from a past life should be a comforting thought; after all, you now have complete control of your life and time. The only restrictions are self-imposed and life is carefree. However, many people are unaware of the impact of retirement on one's psyche. In addition to financial preparations, there are so many other housekeeping issues to attend, that a person may become stressed or overwhelmed by the process.

Someone once stated that retirement preparations should begin from the first day of employment. This seems farfetched and difficult to perceive, but it may be practical. Change interrupts one's life and tosses the comfort zone far away. Most people tend to function more effectively when there is a routine and shudder when the parameters are removed. Fear and uncertainty can replaced calm and order, leading to chaos. It does not have to be this way; so stop, relax, breathe and read the following suggestions that can assist in your EMBRACING CHANGES.

Embracing Changes

1. Allow yourself to feel the changes.

2. Embrace change with positivity.

3. Begin to make plans for your retirement.

   - Start thinking about days without agendas
   - Fine tune your financial plans
   - Beef up community activities of choice
   - Don't forget to make time for your generations.

4. Guide yourself through the physical, emotional, mental, spiritual and cognitive experiences.

5. Change can be painful and difficult, so keep a great attitude about it.

   - Plan ways to make the best of each day
   - Community/volunteer activities

- Spontaneous days

6. Join a support group – if there isn't one, start one. Examples of support groups include:

- Empowered retired men/women
- Bridge/games, club
- Retirement survival/support
- Widows/widower club
- Men support
- Menopause support

7. Begin to think and prepare for the other transition of life – DEATH, and more importantly, ETERNITY.

Change is inevitable; no one (thing) remains the same forever. Learning to embrace change is more challenging. Begin the transformation by mentally preparing to transition through every stage you may traverse. Remember, a positive attitude and a meaningful legacy, can go a long way.

Point to Ponder:

Change is inevitable.

Get ready!

Notes of Reflection

Take A Turn with Self

Dear Readers,

Many of you would recall playing childhood games such as, hopscotch; jump rope and marbles, where everyone waited his/her turn to compete. All it meant was everyone deserved an opportunity to show the others his/her skills and proficiency in said games. Playing these games provided great physical exercises, as well as a chance to bond socially and emotionally.

Similarly, to the childhood games that are archaic today, but we relished so much, we must learn to "take a turn with self." The objective here is to do something beneficial and gratifying for self, while assessing your current life status.

In the popular 1980's hit, "It's my Turn, written by Carole Bayer Sager, and performed by Diana Ross, the lyrics read:

"I can't cover up my feelings in the name of Love, Or play it safe

For a while that was easy. And if living for myself Is what
I'm guilty of,
Go on and sentence me, I'll still be free.

"It's my turn, to see what I can see.
I hope you'll understand, this time's just for me.
Because it's my turn, with no apologies.
I've given up the truth to those I've tried to please.
But Now – It's my turn if I don't have all the answers,
At least I know, I'll take my share of chances.
Ain't no use in holding on when nothing stays the same.
So, I'll let it rain, cause the rain aint gonna hurt me,
And I'll let you go, though I know it won't be easy.

It's my turn, with no more room for lies.
For years I've seen my life through someone else's eyes.
And now it's my turn to try and find my way.
And if I should get lost, at last, I'll own today.
It's my turn. Yes, it's my turn.
Because it's my turn, to turn and say goodbye, I sure
would like to know.

That you're still on my side. It's my turn to start from number one,
Trying to undo some damage that's been done.
But now it's my turn, to reach and touch the sky.
No one's gonna say at least I didn't try.
It's my turn………"

Recognizing that it is your turn requires several tools: First and foremost, take stock of your current position. It doesn't matter how you got here; this is your reality. *Are you happy with this disposition?* This "turn" must be inward. Take a spiritual inventory: - devotions, prayers, meditations – Spend time with God.

Take a mental inventory: - readings, academic advancements, extra classes.

Take an emotional inventory: - Be at peace, forgive, express feelings, communicate, access belongingness, develop self-worth and healthy relationships.

Take a physical inventory: - Is the weight where you desire, have you established the exercise routine; are you eating everything in moderation?

Secondly, draw the line between where you are and where you aspire to be. Set goals to bridge this gap. Goals are small steps that you have designed. They should be tapered to your specification, to meet your standards. Goals should be S.M.A.R.T *(specific, measurable, achievable, relevant and timebound)*. Block out everybody else' wishes for you and concentrate on self.

Thirdly, clean house, both literally and figuratively. Clean the closets and cupboards of your house and get rid of everything you can't fit, don't like, don't wear, don't eat, haven't cooked, or don't need. Clean your surroundings by getting rid of all the toxic people in your life. Anyone who doesn't advance your cause or advance your life, is a cobweb. Sweep them all away.

Fourthly, turn your words around to speak positively. Speak words of affirmation over your life and the lives of your children. Affirmations mean you are reminding yourself of all you are worth and about which you feel good.

Fifthly, if you don't already have new and meaningful relationships, cultivate them. This is important to provide you with a strong support system and people who are on your side. Good relationships build a hedge around and encourage realistic views.

Sixthly, contract to spend at least ten (10) minutes alone, daily. This is time for you to do whatever you want to: rejoice, cry, meditate, think, stare, laugh, dote, run, hide, etc. Do whatever you want to do.

Remember:

- **Live in the present.**

  The past is gone.
  The future is a dream.
  We only have here and now.

- **Celebrate happy moments.**

  That special time in the day that means so much to you.

- **Laugh haughtily, cry passionately.**

  Sleep in that new lingerie.
  Wear that new underwear.
  Eat in that new china in the living room cabinet.
  Have juice in that Lennox wine glass.

- Sit in the living room chair and place your feet on the coffee table.
- Travel to someplace that you have never been.
- Cook a favorite meal and eat all of it.
- Walk around in your bedroom naked.
- Have sex on the rug.
- Dye your hair an eccentric color.
- Appreciate others.
- Appreciate life.
- Appreciate you.

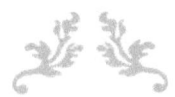

Point to Ponder: It is time to turn on you.

Notes of Reflection

What color is the mask you are wearing?

Dear Readers,

On a trip to Paris, France a few years ago, my daughters and I visited several tourist booths, with a view of securing souvenirs. My younger daughter was drawn to a quaint, picturesque store that had a great selection, from which to choose. It was also a delight to discover that the store owner spoke English.

In the corner of a lower-level shelf, sat an array of trinkets of bright colors. Knowing my younger daughter and her proclivity for 'different,' it came as no surprise that there was an attraction here. On the far end of the shelf, sat a bright pink mask, which she insisted she had to have. The mask was beautifully decorated with bling, and reasonably priced; but I had a difficult time deciphering its necessity. She fell in love with the mask, placed it on her face, boasted of how great she looked in it, purchased it and moved on. Upon arriving home, she placed the mask on a desk in her room as decoration; and that is where it continues to sit.

One definition of mask, labels it "a manner of expression, that hides one's true character or feelings; a pretense." Masks are sometimes worn at events as costumes, keeping others guessing about the identity of their wearers. They prevent others from being able to look into the eyes, which can give a quick glimpse into the soul. They show the world what we want it to see; outward beauty and happiness, while often concealing inner turmoil.

Everyone wears a mask, at some time or another. Some people wear masks of happiness, togetherness, holiness, and perfection; while others wear masks of unkindness, neediness and destitution. These masks show others the part of self that is generally accepted and keeps anyone from knowing who people are truly. Masks allow us to be accepted in a way that brings less attention. The perplexing truth, however, is, very few people can identify masks worn by others.

Being transparent is difficult. Moreover, it is scary, as it determines one's acceptance into a select crowd. Who wants to hear about your troubles? The reality is, to show pain prevents you from being admired. Showing pain labels you as damaged goods, troubled and unattractive, keeping others away from you; thereby promoting isolation; hence, the reason for adorning masks. Wearing masks avoid judgements, condemnation, and exposure to just how messed up we may be. To get a literal picture of a mask, imagine seeing someone whose face looks flawless with make up; then stopping by his/her home, unannounced, when there is no time to apply the layers of foundation and creams. What a sight!! I think you get the picture. There is an ongoing question, **what color mask are you wearing today?**

Masks are usually disrobed in the comfort of homes and dwelling places, where it is safe and harmless to do so. Sometimes, they may come off, slightly, outside of the comfort zones; but if there is a feeling of discomfort, they are quickly placed back on faces. Taking off and placing on masks, is a daunting, tiring task.

There are many hurting people around. Many of them are reaching out for help, but their cries are going unheard. They show us their needs in many ways, they want to totally remove the masks, but we are so often caught up in our stuff, we miss the clues. They want to be believed, loved, HELPED, and accepted; but they get little reception, forcing them to bottle up what they are going through. As they continue stuffing their bags with issues, eventually, the bags, which have limited capacities, explode!

Do me and you a favor, slowly begin removing pieces of your mask, gradually becoming more comfortable showing your true self and getting your needs met. By the same time, encourage others to begin removing their masks and reach out to help them, as you are helping yourself. Ultimately, we will all commence taking off our masks, being assured, that there is another bare face waiting to embrace and be embraced. Take off that mask and sit it on the shelf.

AskDoctorPam – About Mental Health

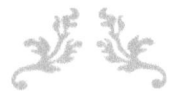

Point to Ponder:

Masks are blinders.

Notes of Reflection

Avoiding medication at your Discretion, is NOT an Option

Dear Readers,

Yesterday, I walked into an office to have a brief conversation with my company's financial director. In the middle of the conversation, I heard a weird moan from her, and she beckoned me to close the door. Immediately following, while sitting at her desk, she went into a full seizure. I knew what was happening and proceeded to speak to her in a slow, methodical and calm manner; the process lasted about three minutes.

At the end of the episode, she explained her situation, diagnosis and prognosis and how she had discontinued her medication. Further, she stated that her situation is exasperated by stress and anxiety. This explanation was so nostalgic, as I recently had the same conversation with a relative, who had been complaining of stomach pains, and excess night anxieties, while refusing to take the prescribed medication.

Panic attacks are generally brought on by excessive anxiety. Anxiety Disorders, though very common, can often be under recognized and undertreated. These disorders are characterized by extreme fretfulness, fear and disturbances in behavior. People experiencing these symptoms, can often feel very afraid and may perceive their imminent deaths.

Anxiety Disorders include ***Social Anxiety Disorder, Selective Mutism, Separation Anxiety, Specific Phobias, Panic Disorder and Generalized Anxiety Disorder (DSM -5)***. Factors that are attributed to Anxiety Disorders include genetics, biopsychosocial factors, trauma and stress. The treatment for Anxiety Disorders, generally include a combination of psychotherapy and pharmacotherapy.

Pharmacotherapy is simply a medical approach to treatment, using drugs; suggesting that the prescribed treatment is done under the guidance of a medical practitioner. It makes good sense to know what your body is absorbing and the side effects that are often present; however, in the words of my friend, B.W., MD, "the need for the medication in your body, usually outweighs the side effects, on your body." Hence, it may be in your best interest to follow the 'fellow' who went to medical school, or at least, have an informed conversation with the same. Moreover, there are 'natural' alternatives to drugs, but these must be discussed, as well. **Avoiding medication at your discretion, is not an option.**

Anxiety, like any other psychological disorder, should always be taken seriously. Even if there is limited understanding of what is being described and felt, we should never minimize what people are experiencing. Someone who is extremely fearful could become harmful to self or others. We must continue to educate ourselves about the things that make and keep us healthy, as well as, what to do if plans go awry. Remember, our physicians care about our wellbeing and only want the best for us. Let us continue to show compassion and sensitivity to all, assisting wherever we are able.

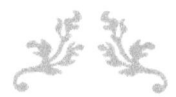

Point to Ponder: Be informed; but use wisdom. It is your life.

Notes of Reflection

Notes of Reflection

Always Check the Intention

Dear Readers,

Knowledge of self is a powerful tool. In fact, the ability to hold self-responsible, while critically examining what is necessary, good and enhancing to healthy development, is a learning curve that many are unable to navigate.

The other day, I placed a quotation on Facebook that garnered some interesting feedback:

"There is a marked difference between negative vibes, and constructive criticism; one refines character, the other breathes schism." - Dr. Pam

While most people agreed with the quotation, a very dear friend suggested that the person on the receiving end of feedback may not be so agreeable. My friend is absolutely correct, so let's have some discussion. I am the first to toot, never let anyone steal your joy; set your pace for the day and stay your course; resist negative energy. My statement, however, does not suggest that we are to live in a vacuum, or that other people's views and perceptions of us, should always be ignored.

Feedback can perhaps be described as a 'necessary evil,' that can have a positive outcome. How paradoxical! Let me then submit, feedback is essential for self-definition. The purpose of feedback is to allow us to see and know how others view our actions and behaviors. Even though most of us (I hope), are intentional with our actions and make every attempt to do the correct things; sometimes we make blunders.

Feedback can be constructive (given in a transparent way to support another), or destructive (specified in a manner to tear down or destroy). Sometimes, the best feedback can be perceived as harmful and difficult to accept. There are two things to think about, when pondering feedback; from whom it comes and the intention of the giver.

We are more inclined to accept feedback from those we consider friends and (most) loved ones. The definition of both groups implies that these are people who care about us and who want to see us develop into our best selves. Thus, no matter how difficult the words, we can find truthful and comforting nuggets to embrace. Moreover, we are usually convinced that people who give us feedback, only want us to tweak the perceptions we have of ourselves and make them even greater. Their aim, is to help 'build' us up, assisting in bringing out the best in us.

There is usually a warm and cozy feeling that one gets when the feedback is honest and helpful. At times, the people who care about us may be harsh in their discourse, so always **check the intention**. When in doubt, ask yourself, if I apply the suggestions given, would they make me a better or bitter person?

Negative vibes can truly lead us to separate ourselves from the transmitters, as such vibes tend to wound our hearts and trouble our spirits.... But constructive words can help to mold our characters, like clay in the hands of a potter.

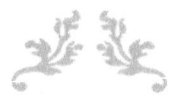

Point to Ponder: "Help me to be the best me and to be open to see what others see."

Notes of Reflection

Notes of Reflection

AskDoctorPam – About Mental Health

Doctors need Doctors, too.

Dear Readers,

The phrase, *'Physician heal thyself,'* taken from the Bible, is often quoted, but do we ever stop to think about what it really means? Simply, the statement reminds us to attend to our faults, in preference to pointing out the faults of others. This is quite an awakening thought, but a sobering prompt to remain vigilant with self-care.

Occupations like mine and others that are similar, are often referred to as the helping profession; so termed, because of the amount of time and methods spent caring for others. These are professions, however, where the 'physicians' are sometimes much wounded and in need of dire care. This is due to the fact that the nature of the work makes it very easy to 'hide.'

I once worked for an outpatient, mental health agency, which utilized the parallel process. The program employs Family Centered Specialists and is based on an evidenced centered model, which emphasizes mimicking the behaviors used in personal life, to the behaviors used with families (patients). In other words, a Specialist who experiences difficulty with confrontation in his/her life; would perhaps never confront a family, with whom s/he works. Or a worker who struggles with timely documentation, perhaps find it difficult holding a family with whom s/he works, accountable. What a great way to keep professional people real! There are still many professionals, however, who continue to slip through the crack.

As practitioners, we need to self-care. This refers to engaging in activities that do not involve elements of our work. Just as we expect the persons for whom we care to be responsible and make good choices; we have to ensure that we are following the same patterns. We should establish boundaries and safeguard that we have a great support system. There should be spiritual and physical activities that are a part of our daily encounters, along with laughter, good company, rest and relaxation. It is oh, so important for us to heal.

Life is already difficult, and people are naturally stressed. We do not need to add any more pressure to our busy schedules; so let us learn to care for self; remember; **DOCTORS NEED DOCTORS, TOO.**

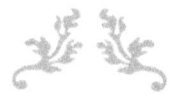

Point to Ponder: I cannot get to you, until I get pass me.

Notes of Reflection

Notes of Reflection

Separation is Never Easy

Dear Readers,

Many children experience Separation Anxiety Disorder, which is a condition that renders them very anxious, when separated from persons to whom they are close. The onset is before the age of 18, but it is usually dominant between the ages of 1 to 4. Older children can also experience this feeling which may be manifested by excess clinginess, staying close to the parent, refusal to sleep at friends' homes, go on errands or attend school. Sometimes physical complaints such as headaches, stomachaches, nausea and vomiting, may accompany.

Realistically speaking, separation is never easy; whether you are parting for a few days, or forever. Saying goodbye, is difficult. Separation means that there is going to be a period when one is not physically present to another. Granted, technology has made this easier, through the years, by applications such as Skype, Zoom, and Facetime, yet it is not the same as reaching across the room and being able to feel the pulse of another.

I was always a wisp when it comes to separating. I have to prepare days in advanced, to approach this really special occasion. I count the days and nights and become more emotional the closer it gets to the appointed time. A big part of this has to do with the fact that I love to be in the company of good people, and often wish this time could last forever. Additionally, with the way that life works, you are never privy to know if you would ever see that individual again.

With this thought in mind, it behooves us to cherish the times and each other. We should spend our lives relishing memories, not reliving regrets. Every moment should be a precious gem to appreciate and remember when we are apart. While in each other's presence, we should ignore the small particles that create schism and do some things without script or agenda. We need to get out of our comfort zones and get into our courage zones.

We should never underestimate what being apart does for some people. This experience can become so overwhelming, it can cause true physical discomfort. Is it any surprise that a strong facet of the grieving process, is the hope of seeing the deceased again? Somehow, this promise brings some level of peace, assurance and eventually, acceptance.

One of the times when separating can be a devastating experience, is when parents move apart. Even when each partner is viewed as the "worst" person ever to have been acquainted, the disseverment of the relationship can have a lasting, sometimes permanent effect on all involved. This is partly due to the fact that people are gregarious by nature and desirous of having long lasting, intimidate ties. When ties are severed; hearts are often broken.

I recently reacquainted with many of my high school classmates from the Class of 1979 of The Government High School. Through the assistance of WhatsApp, and, the efforts of a few skilled people, we have been reunited, after 37 years. One thing is for certain, we will never be estranged again!

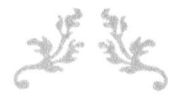

Point to Ponder:

Separate, don't

dissipate.

Notes of Reflection

Notes of Reflection

AskDoctorPam – About Mental Health

I Even role play with Myself

Dear Readers,

Some time ago, I was asked by a curious student if it is fine to talk to oneself. I told her that I did not know a better way to stay in touch with self. I informed her that not only do I talk to myself, but I answer myself and I even role play with myself.

It is a fact that it does not matter who we are, there are time in our lives we experience feelings of fear, doubt, loneliness, and grief. These feelings are usually associated with pain and anguish. Sometimes the pain can become so overwhelming, that it may require some strong refocusing to get back on the path. The most vulnerable times tend to occur when we are alone. This is the time when self-talk is most beneficial.

Self-talk is that personal conversation that you have with yourself. The paragraphs can be rehearsed, structured, and recited; or they can be impulsive, pure and extemporaneous. Ideally, self-talks are motivational, inspiring, uplifting, confirming and positive. Conversely, self-talks can be deflating, destructive, guilt ridden and negative. Some people learn to self-talk in a formal manner, while others learn through experience. Whatever "talks" one has with self, strengthens the belief system, and are greatly related to the action (s) that follow.

Self-talk is particularly significant when one experiences difficult times in his/her life. No matter how much others are concerned with our wellbeing, no one is around us every minute of our lives; there are many hours that we spend alone. It is usually during these times that self-doubt, anxiety and fear are pervasive. No human being can define or experience our despair, which often results in panic. In the natural, we are with ourselves, by ourselves and this can be a scary time, especially, if we don't know ourselves.

Hence, we have to do for ourselves, what no one else can; we have to believe in our strengths and abilities. We should be able to bring ourselves to a place of peace, calm and hope using self-=talk. The aim, therefore, is to make self-talks so encouraging, that we can believe our words. Here are seven ways to perfect self-talks:

1. Never forget that we can only do some things from self, but all things through God.

2. Develop a self-talk strategy, before there is crisis.

3. Make your self-talk with positive, believable words.

4. Talk to yourself daily. Listen to yourself, as well.

5. Practice your self-talk in the mirror.

6. Study motivational quotes.

7. Begin and end all talks with gratitude.

In case you are wondering what role playing is and how it works, it is a higher form of self-talk, where you can become completely transparent with self, and you are able to walk in the shoes of another. These types of self-talk usually culminate in forgiveness.

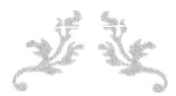

Point to Ponder: The more I talk to myself, the better I am able to understand me.

Notes of Reflection

Notes of Reflection

AskDoctorPam – About Mental Health

Live your Most Authentic Life

Dear Readers,

"The privilege of a lifetime is to become who you truly are." -Carl Jung

Several months ago, a relative of mine embarked upon a journey of a life time: she wanted to lose some weight and begin a healthier choice track. Ten months later, she is down 10 dress sizes and has lost about 70 pounds. In a recent Facebook post, she retorted about how she has been criticized for her efforts and told many disparaging things. She could not understand why everyone was not happy for her accomplishment. I commended her for the bravery and tenacity exhibited and encouraged her to live her most authentic life.

Authentic living is being the best of you. It does not deal with the imitation of who we think we should be, or have been told we should be; it is who we have allowed ourselves to become. There is no "should" in authenticity. Authenticity involves transparency, hard work, tweaking, trials and errors. When I was in graduate school, one of my psychology professors used to talk about, "peeling away the layers of the onions." This is symbolic of getting rid of the façades and showing the true person. Authenticity consists of being comfortable with self and acceptance of self-truth. There are three very important concepts to consider when dealing with authentic living: values/beliefs, past life and dynamism.

Each of us has a set of beliefs that were taught to us, or that we have developed through the years. In order to be the best person that we can, we have to examine our values. These values have to truly be a part of who we are and what we accept as truth. For example, if we were raised with and believe in regular church attendance and have been exposed to Christian truths, but have found that we seldom attend church, and we are sharing a common space with a person who is not our spouse, this is not authentic living. In order to make this truth relevant to our system of authenticity, we would have to correct the inconsistencies in this thinking, or eliminate this belief as one of ours. Authentic living, demands us to believe in what we do and do what we believe.

A second major component in authenticity is dealing with the past. We have to arrest all the thoughts and feelings that keep us tied to the past. Anything that serves as an anchor to keep us unable to move forward, will keep us in the past. The past is gone and can no longer be lived. It can serve as a reminder of current growth and motivate us to move onward, but never to keep us bound. In instances where we are unable to 'shake' the past, we should seek professional help to assist us. Authentic living requires us to live in the here and now.

A third component to living authentically, is the ability to evolve as a person. This includes the process of experiencing new learning, checking our current status and making appropriate adjustments. There are new trends and ideas that change daily. This is not to suggest that it is necessary to make daily changes, but rather to accept things around us that help to bring a more defined view of who we purport to be. Authentic living connotes that life is dynamic. Authentic living was never meant to be simple. It, however, separates the real from the fakers and holds all, who subscribe to it, accountable.

"The good life is a process, not a state of being. It is a direction not a destination."
- Carl Rogers

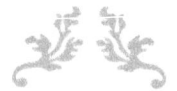

Point to Ponder:

Life is too short to live in untruth.

Notes of Reflection

Notes of Reflection

AskDoctorPam – About Mental Health

Walls of Fear

Dear Readers,

As a noun, **fear** is described as an emotion that is caused when one believes someone, or something is dangerous, presents a threat, or can cause pain. As a verb, **fear** means to be afraid of someone, or something that is likely to be dangerous, painful or dangerous. Either way, fear can become overpowering, almost to the point of paralysis; leading to psychological and physiological distress. Success comes, when you are able to conquer your fears and move on with your life. My niece Jani, granted me permission to print a poem she scribed, when asked to explore her fears. Read it carefully, as some things are implied, not stated; leaving the reader to fill in the blanks…..*be fearful!*

Walls of Fear written by Jani Pierre

Some walls are unbreakable, called the walls of fear,

Like losing a loved one, or speaking in front of your peers.

Fear of being humiliated, fear of being shamed,

Mills

If these walls are not broken, who am I to blame?

Fear can be destructive, they tear you up inside,

Fear is like a roller coaster, taking you for the ride,

Why are my fears so controlling, telling me what to do?

Just let me have my freedom, am I a slave to you?

Fear is like a bully, and you are the outcast,

It is like a lion coming at you, moving way too fast.

Fear is our challenge, will we break the walls?

Will we overcome them, or stumble and fall?

As the wind blows, the windmill spins, and spins,

Adapting to new settings, as though life just begins.

New faces and new places, alone and brand new,

Heart beating like a drum, no idea what to do.

Little by little I open up, like a flower starts to bloom,

The flower starts to close back up, entering the room.

Silence fills the atmosphere, as quiet as day,

The noise begins to amplify, still nothing to say.

As the flower reopens at ease, it starts to multiply,

AskDoctorPam – About Mental Health

From one flower to the first, why were you so shy?

Like in spring, the flower starts to blend,

Turns into a garden, everyday a new friend.

Day by day I gaze about, thinking of the past,

Nine years now ten approaching, time went by so fast.

You were here but now you're gone, on to a better place,

Wish that you could be right here, just to see your face.

Tears shed, grief comes, sadness and despair,

The absence of your mellow voice, sadly fills the air.

Even though the sun is out, it has never been so dark.

Blackness fills the empty space, without you there is no spark. Gave me life and robbed of yours, from sickness that was there, Asked the Lord to take you home, the pain you could not bear.

For every life there is a death, a lesson overcame,

The windmill prevailed over the wind, life never remains the same!

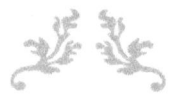

Point to Ponder:

Have no fear, God is here!

Notes of Reflection

Notes of Reflection

AskDoctorPam – About Mental Health

The Bigger Storm, After the Storm

Dear Readers,

I can vividly recall the death of my third brother; it was like yesterday, and a most painful experience. The dreadful phone call that woke me from a deep sleep as I laid relaxing after studying eight grueling hours for a mid-term exam, is etched in my memory. I was a third-year university student at the time, enjoying my college life. This death which interrupted my peaceful life was an intruder.

Moving about my business, I traveled to New Providence to commence funeral plans. While assisting his wife with clothes and cemetery selections, I never made plans to grieve. Keeping busy with so many tasks, was my escape from reality. On the day of the funeral when his body was returned to the earth, all I can recall is being carted off by family members who later informed me that I had liquids flowing from every orifice in my body, enter- **POSTTRAUMATIC STRESS**.

I arise at 5 a.m. every day to exercise. This routine includes placing the television on channel 11, where I could adhere to the announcements and tune into a prayer ritual, for the *"Hour of Prayer."* One day, I made a startling discovery. It appeared as if almost seven out of every ten death notices or funeral announcements, on the television, were of elderly residents. These were people who resided on an island, that has recently experienced a hurricane. I immediately thought, we may be so consumed with replacing houses destroyed, that we may have inadvertently forgotten the needs of the two most vulnerable groups, the children and the elderly. This may have placed us amid the BIGGER storm, after the storm.

Posttraumatic stress is a serious disorder that is characterized by developing symptoms following exposure to an extreme traumatic stressor (Hurricanes, earthquakes, etc.), involving direct personal experience of an event that involves actual or threatened death or serious injury, or threat to physical integrity; or witnessing a traumatic death or injury of another; or learning of unexpected death, injury, or harm of a family member (DSM 5). The disorder can render feelings of avoidance with any thought or feeling associated with the event, or avoiding people, places or activities associated with the event, inability to recall, diminished participation in usual activities; feelings of detachment or estrangement from others; inability to have loving feelings and the inability to foresee a future or future plans.

Additionally, other physical symptoms can include problems with sleep, irritability or outbursts of anger, difficulty concentrating, hyper vigilance and exaggerated startle response. Intense fear and helplessness may also be experienced. The trauma may be persistently re-experienced. The disorder is called Post traumatic because it occurs weeks and months after the trauma.

In the recovery process of a traumatic natural disaster, we must ensure that our citizens are cared for from a holistic point of view. Everyone, who was exposed to the traumatic effects of this storm, should be involved in weekly therapy sessions. In doing so, let us not forget the children and elderly. While children tend to be more resilient, the senior citizens among us may be more reserved. They are consumed with living the rest of their lives as simply and meaningful as possible. A big part of this wish is to live in the communities that they have called home for so many years, with their daily routines, enjoying the moments.

Now, however, many of them have been displaced and may have developed a great sense of despair, feeling scared, concerned and uncertainty. Moreover, if someone is not monitoring these feelings and paying attention to all their needs, the elderly may bottle up these feelings and "pine" themselves out of this world. Hence, if you have to care for your parents, children, or anyone for that matter, who were victims of a catastrophe, please talk to them daily. If you are unable to secure therapy for them, the following steps may be followed:

1. Allow them to talk (vent). This validates their feelings.

2. Listen to the stories as often as they tell them. Show them love and treat them with kindness

(don't make them feel as if their presence is an inconvenience in your life).

3. Ask questions about their care (assess food intake, comfort, and physical/mental health)

4. Ensure that they seek regular medical care.

5. Replicate the environment, as much as possible, to what they were use.

6. Ensure that some routine is done daily (regular activities such as reading, watching television, or listening to the radio, church activities, etc.). This will increase mental acuity.

7. Allow them to participate in their care and desires. Treat them with dignity.

8. Check in with them regularly, asking what is fine and what can be improved.

9. Validate their feelings and discuss goals.

10. Reassure them that things will be fine and tell them how much they mean to you. This will strengthen their faith, hopes and dreams and give them a reason to live.

Let us continue to take care of each other.

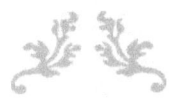

Point to Ponder:

The elderly, we won't have with us always.

Notes of Reflection

Panic Attack

Dear Readers,

On Wednesday past, I was driving home from work, when I was led to telephone a relative. She answered the phone in an excitable manner and this prompted me to ask if all was well. She disclosed that she was currently in the emergency room of a local hospital, explaining how she felt she was dying. According to her, she had not been regularly sleeping, was feeling overwhelmed, dizziness, shortness of breath, pain in her arms and chest pains. She had an Electrocardiogram (heart test), which was normal, and was awaiting the results from a blood panel. I encouraged her to take deep breaths and patiently wait; I further informed her, that based on the symptoms described and my knowledge of her present situation, it sounded like she was experiencing an acute panic attack.

Panic attacks are generally brought on by excessive anxiety. Anxiety Disorders, though very common, can often be under recognized and undertreated. These disorders are characterized by extreme fretfulness, fear and disturbances in behavior. People experiencing these symptoms can often feel very afraid and may perceive their imminent deaths.

Anxiety Disorders include Social Anxiety Disorder, Selective Mutism, Separation Anxiety, Specific Phobias, Panic Disorder and Generalized Anxiety Disorder (DSM -5). Factors that are attributed to Anxiety Disorders include genetics, biopsychosocial factors, trauma and stress. The treatment for Anxiety Disorders, generally include a combination of psychotherapy and pharmacotherapy.

The relative described above, is currently pursuing an intense academic program and it is approaching the end of the fall semester. She has several scholarly papers, presentations and final examinations, that are all due within the next three weeks. She is extremely stressed and has been given a strict prescription to ensure a successful semester's end. Her symptoms were not life threatening, even though it felt that way to her.

Anxiety, like any other psychological disorder, should always be taken seriously. Even if there is limited understanding of what is being described and felt, we should never minimize what people are experiencing. Someone who is extremely fearful could become harmful to self or others. We must continue to educate ourselves about the things that make and keep us healthy, as well as, what to do if things go awry. Let us continue to show care and sensitivity to all, assisting wherever we are able, especially in this post storm era.

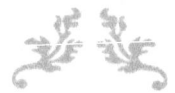

Point to Ponder:

Sometimes we must slow down to speed up.

Notes of Reflection

Notes of Reflection

Courage to change the things I can

Dear Readers,

Addiction is a serious phenomenon. It suggests that one has limited control over certain persons, things, activities, or substances in his/her life. Addiction is serious because it can rob you of the main essence of life and leave you feeling useless and defenseless. It is difficult to live with an addiction and even more difficult to cure one. The main mantra for an addict, is the Serenity Prayer:

God grant me the serenity
To accept the things I cannot change;
Courage to change the things I can;
And wisdom to know the difference.

Living one day at a time;
Enjoying one moment at a time;
Accepting hardships as the pathway to peace;
Taking, as He did, this sinful world
As it is, not as I would have it;
Trusting that He will make all things right

If I surrender to His Will;
So that I may be reasonably happy in this life
And supremely happy with Him
Forever and ever in the next.
Amen.

Reinhold Neibuhur 1892-1971

One of the greatest lines in this prayer, and perhaps the most humbling to an addict, is the process of accepting things that he/she is unable to change. This is a difficult concept for any person, especially when so many seem to be obsessed with making changes to everything; particularly to circumstances that manifest as undesirable and painful. Dealing with such circumstances can prove to be taxing on all facets of life.

Some elections in the United States have left many feeling this way. Man seems relentless in his pursuit to be able to know and predict things. When things appear to be going contrary to what he believes they should be, he feels restless, confused, and determined to find the logic in the situation. Somethings, however, defy logic. God in his wisdom, never gifted any ONE person with the ability to know and understand EVEYHING; had he done this, that person (s) would have challenge him for his sovereignty. When things happen that seem beyond your control, good, bad, or indifferent, accept the results as final. Trust God with the way forward. Deal with the things you can change and change them!

I have lived long enough to know these four things; God does not need my permission to do anything, things are never what they seem, it isn't over until it is over, and flesh will fail me. Therefore, I live my life by this simple philosophy: Nothing in life surprises me; I may be disappointed, but never surprised. I have learned to accept life's challenges, despite how difficult they may be, learn the lesson from each experience, change the things I can and must and move on.

This is not to suggest that there are not temporary setbacks or pain. In truth, sometimes the pain seems unbearable and eternal, but I insist on seeing it as intermittent paralysis, believing if I push through it with the right attitude, intentions and determination, I will walk again. This strength comes from my faith in God and his promise to finish the work he has begun in me. The reality being, no matter how we squabble, we will never be able to change some things.

In the treatment of addicts, the goal is to get them to move from denial to acceptance and the first objective in most treatment programs, is to encourage persons to admit that they are powerless over certain things; that way, they would resist the temptation in believing that everything is under their control. They are taught to expend the energy, exacting the things that they can and leaving the rest to a higher power; that speaks to *"the wisdom in knowing the difference."*

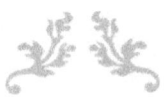

Point to Ponder:

Got Serenity?

Notes of Reflection

AskDoctorPam – About Mental Health

Living with Schizophrenia

Dear Readers,

Roy is a 46 – year old black divorced male who is slim, weighing 116 pounds and stands 5'8" tall. Roy has no children and was born in a small settlement on a southern island in the Bahamas; Roy lives in New Providence. Roy's parents hail from a larger island in the Caribbean. Roy refused to give any details about his father, only stating that when his family migrated to the Bahamas, his father did not accompany them. "I have no idea what happened to him, and I don't really care. He left us when I was very young, and I never asked my mom to tell us what happened. Who cares?"

Roy's mom works in a clothing store, and she just celebrated her 71st birthday. Roy has an older brother, Jay and a younger sister, Marla. Jay lives on a neighboring island and sees Roy about twice a year; Marla lives close by, "but hates me and I hate her; she is a mean witch, mean to me and to her children. I can't stand her." Roy has no children, "and I don't intend to have any. With me being sick and all, there is no need to have children. They couldn't help me any."

Roy has spent the last 16 years in and out of psychiatric hospitals because of his problems. He tells the psychiatrist, "I came to you because I was told to. The fires in my head started again. I can't get rid of them. And I itch all over. It's like little things are running all over my body. Look at my arms (he shows arms which are scratched raw). I also have some breathing problems."

Roy sweats profusely, even when it is cool outside, he makes poor eye contact throughout his sessions, frequently looking at the walls or out of the window. Many times, he stares at the radio or telephone, sometimes at a flowering plant on the desk. Roy is living with Schizophrenia. (Adapted from Getzfeld, 2004).

Schizophrenia is a mental disorder which does not discriminate; it occurs in people of all cultures and walks of life. The most salient feature of this disorder is the loss of contact with reality. Some of the symptoms include distortions in perception, thinking, action, sense of self and manner in relating to others (Hooley, 2014).

Common terms associated with schizophrenia are delusions (disturbances in thought) and hallucinations (seeing, hearing, touching, and feeling things that seem real, but are not there).

Historically, there were several subtypes of Schizophrenia, however, today, the new classification is Schizophrenia Spectrum Disorders (Schizophreniform, Schizoaffective, Delusional, Brief Psychotic Disorders) (DSM-5, 2013). Clinical significance includes, unreal and illogical beliefs, highly elaborated and organized into a coherent, though delusional framework, flat or inappropriate emotions, disorganized speech, and disorganized behaviors, and exaggerated motor signs that reflect great excitement or stupor (DSM-5, 2013).

Research suggests that schizophrenia has a strong genetic component (runs in families), but can be perpetuated by environmental factors (stress, living conditions, etc). There are many people living with schizophrenia around the world. Schizophrenia must be diagnosed by trained personnel, namely a psychiatrist, physician, or clinical psychologist. Schizophrenia is usually treated with pharmacological (medicine), therapeutic and psychosocial approaches. However, it is most effectively treated when these approaches work in tandem. Family and community support are paramount. If you suspect that you are living with this disorder, please visit a local hospital. Be informed!

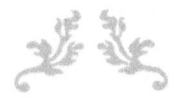

Point to Ponder:

Living with knowledge, beats dying of ignorance.

Notes of Reflection

Letters to Dr. Pam

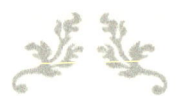

The names in each letter represented on the pages to follow have been changed to reflect their initials only.

Homelessness

Dear Dr. Pam,

I am a law-abiding citizen who pays her dues. I am, however, concerned about the number of homeless persons who walk around our streets, aimlessly. These people are extremely unkempt, smelly and beggars! I am afraid that they will chase our tourists away making things worst in these already challenging economic times. *Whose problem is this?*

-S.K.

Dear S.K.,

THESE PEOPLE and THIS PROBLEM should be all our concern, as they are a part of us. The interesting fact of the matter is that many homeless people have homes and caring family members and support systems. The issue is, however, many of them do not want to be confounded to a home.

In some countries, homeless people have voluntarily vacated mental health facilities. Hence, research seems to suggest, that there is sometimes a relationship between homeless people and mental disorders; most notably, Schizophrenia (a mental disorder that presents with a split between thoughts and emotions, personality disturbance and accompanied by delusions, hallucinations, and irrational fears), which can render one vulnerable enough to wander. Medication and therapy assist with decreasing the symptoms. There is usually a barrage of reasons why this course of action is not followed.

Some people are homeless because economic circumstance rendered them that way. They honestly have nowhere to go and seek alternative living arrangements, such as shelters. Many roam the streets soliciting funds and food from whomever would give. Being homeless is not a crime, but some homeless people commit criminal activities.

Homeless people are generally harmless unless they feel threatened. Under such circumstances, they may defend themselves. What you and I can do is discourage their habits by not supporting them and encouraging them to return home. For those who may have loved ones on the streets, go and look for them, with a view of helping them to get the help that they need. There are also housing facilities that cater to the care of this population.

-Dr. Pam

Point to Ponder: Homelessness is no respect of person.

Am I Socially Fit?

Dear Dr. Pam,

I have not been diagnosed with, but I think I suffer from Social Anxiety. I am not currently employed and feel that this disorder may be a part of the problem. I avoid people at all cost and general social settings. I would like to know if there is anything I can do to help my situation, without becoming a financial burden on my family?

-A.B.

Dear A. B.,

I always find the field of self-diagnosing very amusing and interesting. Social Anxiety (diagnostically defined as Social Phobia) is a disorder marked with a persistent fear of social situations, that can cause embarrassment. Almost immediately, an anxiety response is triggered causing discomfort for the individual. Therefore, such social situations are avoided. This disorder can occur in children and adults. It is a serious disorder that can interfere with an individual's day to day, family, and occupational activities. Suffice it to say, the social life is almost nonexistent.

However, caution must be taken to ensure that other conditions are ruled out before this diagnosis is made. As with any other issue, a professional should be consulted to ensure proper diagnosis and a relevant treatment path.

Since something is impeding your upward mobility, find a trusted therapist and work through this issue. Discuss this concern with your family members and solicit their support. Once you are on a path of recovery, your life should become enhanced. People who suffer from social phobias can lead regular lives with proper treatment.

-Dr. Pam

Dear Readers,

If you work long and difficult hours like me, I am certain you must long for times when you can relax and enjoy yourself and others. Begin by asking yourself, "Am I socially fit?" Here are some pointers to improve your social life:

1. Find time to do something that you enjoy, with no agenda.

2. Treat yourself with a special token whenever you are paid.

3. Go out occasionally and meet at least one new person.

4. Play games with your spouse, children, or friends. Act childish.

5. Rekindle relationships.

6. Laugh at your jokes.

7. Join a book or civil club.

8. Join your neighbors and plan a block party.

Point to Ponder: Your social life, like every other aspect of you, needs to be cultivated.

Your Parents Already Know About Your Lifestyle

Dear Dr. Pam,

Can you explain why school children are cutting themselves? I am a young woman, and I can't understand this behavior.

- RDK

Dear RDK,

This is sad but true. Some teenagers (particularly) are exhibiting what is known as Self Injurious Behaviors or Self-Mutilation. Although this behavior can occur with males, more females are victims. People generally cut themselves as a method of dealing with issues. The idea of cutting is symbolic of "slicing away" at the pain in their lives. This pain represents all issues that they deem difficult and stressful.

Common areas of the body susceptible to being cut include the upper parts and insides of the arm/wrist and the thigh. Often, long sleeved garments are worn to camouflage the scars. Mutilators sometimes cut until they bleed, and the production of the incision produces a 'rush' and a release of pressure and pain. They view this activity as productive, not painful. The method of cutting varies from person to person, but usually long horizontal strokes are created. Razors, knives, compasses, pens, pencils or any other sharp objects are the tools of choice, and these tools are usually kept hidden. Mutilators can bleed to death or even sever body parts. Cutting is most often done during quiet times in isolation.

Even though this may seem like an unusual manner of problem solving, it is real and deadly. Therefore, if you know someone who mutilates self, encourage that person to talk to a parent, school counselor clergy, or a trusted adult. Parents, if you suspect your child is cutting, examine the body parts mentioned and immediately seek professional help.

-Dr. Pam

Dear Dr. Pam,

I am a male college student abroad who is a practicing homosexual. I am very distraught about my situation as I am 'in the closet.' I could never have this conversation with my parents and worse, live in our homophobic hometown. I must, however, return home. Please help!
-ABC

Dear ABC,

Thank you for sharing such sensitive information with me. I would suggest that you spend some time in meditation and decide with what information you want to proceed. You already have a sense of the hometown's general perception of your lifestyle, and you appear to need its blessings. Speak with someone you trust and bounce ideas and suggestions off that individual. Arrange a meeting with your parents and tell them what you want them to know. You may be surprised to discover that your parents already know about your lifestyle.

-Dr. Pam

Dear Reader,

Here are three things you can do with your family that do not cost you a penny; however, your gains are beyond wealth:

1. Eat at least one meal together.
2. Talk walks as a family.
3. Have a family fun night every week.

Point to Ponder:

Be observant and gentle.

Grieve Completely

Dear Dr. Pam,

Why does it seem that some black people view therapy as a "white people" thing?

-J.D.

Dear J.D.,

This is such an astute observation, and unfortunately a true one. Historically, many black families used the African tradition of having problems resolved within the family. The elders of the village would gather and decide solutions for social, marital and emotional issues. Many African cultures still do this.

In the not so distant past, remnants of this problem solving methods were still active. The extended family played a vital role in ensuring that members of the family were stable and assisted in problem solving, for a healthier family.

Today, people appear more independent and empowered and choose a myriad of ways to resolve issues. Traditional therapeutic approaches have not been embraced, predominantly because these approaches are not always understood. In some black cultures to seek emotional assistance from trained personnel, such as, a psychologist or psychiatrist is still tabooed.

Only people who understand the valuable contributions, processes and procedures of therapy endorse the services. Ironically, people who have come to terms that they need therapeutic services and seek them out, are viewed as being in positions to learn how to make healthier choices for themselves. After all, the first step to solving a problem is admitting that you have a problem. I guess many "white" people have realized this.

- Dr. Pam

Dear Dr. Pam,

What advice would you give to a young widow about dating? What would you consider to be an appropriate time to start dating again?

-A.J.

Dear A.J.,

Like anything, readiness is a determinant in everything. There is no hard and fast rule about returning to the "love race," but ensuring that all issues associated with the former relationship are sorted. If there is unfinished emotional business, it has to be completely resolved before embarking upon any new ventures. Grieve cautiously, critically and completely.

-Dr. Pam

Point to Ponder: Clearing away of old things, makes more space for new things.

AskDoctorPam – About Mental Health

A Letter to our Mummy

Dear Readers,

I was going through my electronic files recently, when I happened upon a letter that was written by two children (male and female, ages 9 and 11, respectively), approximately four years ago, upon the death of their mother. It reads as follows:

A LETTER TO OUR MUMMY

Dear Mummy,

We love you and we'll always keep you in our hearts. You were a good mother and we will never be apart. We still care for you and love you dearly. We will continue to pray like you taught us to do. You taught us to trust God and to live holy. We hope you feel better in your new home, where you will never be sick or alone. We hope you remember us each day, as we remember you. Thanks for loving us and teaching us to be thankful, as we MUST TRUST GOD.

Good Night, Mummy!
Love Always.

Death is a difficult concept with which to deal, and it can be even more difficult when one does not quite understand its purpose. A part of this perceived confusion is the fact that death seems so final.

When a loved one passes away, the survivors are usually overcome with a barrage of emotions. The grieving process can last from a few weeks to several years. It is important that there is a grieving period. This period is tantamount to learning how to cope and survive without the deceased.

Children need to have an opportunity to grieve, and understanding two concepts, chronological age, and development stage, will assist in this process. We know that infants and toddlers do not intellectually comprehend the death of a loved one, but they realize that someone important is gone, as they miss certain things, such as the person's voice or touch. We also know that preschoolers through first graders experience difficulty with the concept of time, thus 'forever' may be viewed as a few hours from now. Usually, it is not until toward the end of first grade through third grade, that there is some understanding of death being final. However, research seems to support the age of nine as the true emergence of understanding the death phenomenon. It is therefore crucial to pay attention to children's responses to death and be prepared to intelligently answer questions asked.

Children's behaviors and actions may vary with the announcement of a death. These may include regressive behaviors (reverting to a younger stage of development), fear, uncertainty, aggressiveness, hearing, seeing and having conversations with the deceased, guilt, worry, sleeplessness, poor appetite, outbursts, or excessive crying. These actions are all acceptable and should only be flagged if they persist for a lengthy period.

Children need consistency and clarity. Euphemisms (daddy is sleeping or gone on a long trip) may confuse them. Acknowledge their concerns, work with them, give them lots of activities and include them (where appropriate) in all the plans. As a caution, children should never be viewed as 'mini adults' and levied with the responsibility of being the man or woman of the house. In the letter above, it is clear that this mother taught her children about death and dying, making it easier for them to deal with her demise. Moreover, the opportunity provided to write a letter to their mother, made them feel a part of the program and commenced the healing process.

-Dr. Pam

Point to Ponder:

Children have feelings, too.

Morning after Pill

Dear Dr. Pam,

I have noticed that I take on the traits of my father (being overly sensitive and emotional); whereas, my sibling, is a brutally honest individual just as my mother. Like my father, I don't care to socialize with people on a regular basis, and I am very introverted.

Even though my siblings and I grew up in the same household, we are like night and day. Can I change my personal persona overtime, or have these characteristics been permanently embedded into my being?

-KDB

Dear KDB,

Many of the popular theories in Psychology place a lot of time in investigating if most of the characteristics that we develop in childhood are permanent and affix, or do we change in predictable and unpredictable ways over the course of our lives? My professional view on this subject is to encourage anyone who wants to make changes in his /her life, to seek the appropriate assistance and do so.

It is very encouraging to know that individuals evaluate themselves, with a view of desiring more for their lives. This is empowerment. May I also add that many of the traits that you have identified are learned; accordingly, they can be unlearned. Take some risks and do some things that are generally a struggle for you, see how you feel and think about them and repeat or discontinue as you deem necessary.

-Dr. Pam

Dear Dr. Pam,

Recently in headline news, several schools in New York have started supplying female students, as young as 14 years, with the "morning after pill." This prevention campaign seeks to reduce the amount of teenage pregnancy. It is safe to say that there is still an alarming amount of teenage pregnancy.

Should every country follow New York's lead in dispensing "morning after pills?" If not, what are other new alternatives to reducing teenage pregnancy?

-VLC

Dear VLC,

I don't like to assume statistics because they look a certain way. Per capita, I do agree that some regions appear to have more teenage mothers than others. To distribute "morning after pills" may work well for New York and we do not know the circumstances. However, I am a proponent of information giving. I think we need to continue talking to our young people on issues of sexuality emphasizing that they always have a choice.

The problem with this is, many adults are uncomfortable with the topic of sex, so how can you teach what you are tensed about learning? Parents should take the initiative in telling their children truths about sexuality; encouraging them to ask questions and come to them when uncertain. Family Life teachers in the schools can reiterate this information, while the church follows the trend.

The fact that the pill is distributed the morning after suggests the level of confusing. It shows that we are not reaching our youth. To arbitrarily dispense "morning after" pills, when the information and decision should have been made the day before, in my opinion is irresponsible.

-Dr. Pam

Point to Ponder: The uniquely colored small fish in the big pond gets a lot of attention too.

Mills

What is the point in Living?

Dear Dr. Pam,

What is the point in living if we are going to die anyway?
-Unknown

Dear Unknown,

Usually when persons ask such seeking questions, they may be experiencing a "dark place;" most notably, depression. If you think you are depressed, I am encouraging you to seek help immediately. You may speak with a counselor, spiritual leader, or go to the emergency room of the nearest hospital.

To answer your question and validate your premise; we begin to die from the moment we are born. However, life is a gift given to us by God. He has a plan for each life. His desire is for us to fulfill the plan. Hence, at this time, you need to validate your existence. Sit somewhere quiet with pen and paper. Divide the paper into two columns. In one column, list all of your contributions to your life to date; this may include completing school, getting a job, etc., anything that advanced the course of your life. In the second column, list all of the plans you have for your life. Then, in the bottom of the page, write all of the limitations you perceive as obstacles to fulfilling your dreams. This exercise should aid you in finding purpose for your life. If you find this assignment difficult to begin or complete, go and see one of the aforementioned persons, immediately.

-Dr. Pam

Dear Dr. Pam,

Growing up in a religious home, we were taught at an early age about sovereignty. This also revolves around the area of choices. Do we truly have choices in our lives and over situations, or is everything preordained?

-Anonymous

Dear Anonymous,

Here are my thoughts. We do know that God is sovereign, which also renders Him omnipresent and omnipotent. When we were created, God gave us the highest order of all species, by virtue of making us with brains that are able to think in logical, rational ways. We have therefore, been given the ability to choose. Free will to man is not an illusion, it is real; and because God is also all knowing, our choices and desires are known by Him. However, He still permits us to make selections.

God has a plan for our lives, but His plan never overrides our will. In respecting His sovereignty, it is wise to seek His guidance in our decisions. He wants us to have an abundant life, so it is not His desire for any one of us to perish, but rather to have the best life ever. Therefore, be governed by His sovereignty and make wise choices. A spiritual leader can expand on this theory, so seek out one.

- Dr. Pam

Sadly, the Church is No Exception

Dear Dr. Pam,

The interviews from members of the public when church elders are involved in legal issues, sometimes leave me ashamed, angry, and disappointed. People in positions of authority should be informed before they speak. Would you please reprint that article on Pedophilia so that our leaders could understand and speak intelligibly?

-T.I.F.

Dear TIF,

With pleasure!

An individual who has sexual attraction for children, is called a Pedophile. Pedophilia is a Sexual and Gender Identity Disorder, which involves any sexual activity of a sixteen-year-old or older individual, with a child who has not reached puberty (usually age 13 or younger). Pedophiles generally have attractions to children of a particular age range, but the attraction can be for males, females, or both. The perpetrators can be family members, friends, or strangers. Such activities can significantly distress or impair the victims' social, occupational, or other important areas of functioning.

The onus is on parents to ensure they know the people with whom they leave their children. However, since parents can't be with their children 24 hours a day, they should equip them with the knowledge of good and evil. Moreover, parents should maintain open and appropriate relationships with their children and talk to them daily, so that they are apprised of concerns in their children's lives.

Pedophiles can be found among any audience, sadly, the church is no exception.

- Dr. Pam

Dear Dr. Pam,

I have watched you over the years. I find you to be sincere, candid, informative, confident, and approachable. I admire and appreciate you. But I am curious. You seemed to be so busy and involved. Where do you go to get your counseling?

- Grateful

Dear Grateful,

Thank you for your kind words. Everyone has issues and psychologists are no exception. I have a very dedicated relationship with God. I spend time daily in prayer and meditation. My support system (comprising family members, friends, and colleagues) is very strong. I own my actions, embrace my strengths and work on my limitations. I am by no means infallible but would like to think that I am well on my way to self-actualizing.

-Dr. Pam

Point to Ponder: One of the greatest flaws of a human being is the unwillingness to take responsibility for his actions.

Author Biography

Dr. Pam is a clinical psychologist, who lives in the Washington, DC area, with her three adult daughters and dog, Teddy Bear. She works with diverse populations, including Individuals with Intellectual Disabilities and as an adjunct university professor. She has over 30 years in the field of mental health and is a sought-after motivational speaker. She was educated in The Bahamas, Jamaica and the United States.

Dr. Pam, through her Damara Mental Health and Educational Services, offers courses and counseling in Crisis, Grief and Bereavement, Individual, Couples,' Marriage and Family Therapy. She is a motivational speaker and consultant, who believes in empowerment to the path of self-discovery.

To contact Author, Dr. Pamula Mills, please:

Visit us Online at:

www.damarahelps.com

Phone:

410-404-4973

E-mail:

askdoctorpam@yahoo.com

damarahelps@gmail.com

References

American Psychiatric Association. (2022). Diagnostical and statistical manual of mental disorders (5th ed., text.rev.).

Butcher, J. N., Hooley, J. M. (2013). Abnormal Psychology. (16 ed.) Pearson.

Getzfeld, A. R. (2004). Essentials of Abnormal Psychology. John Wiley & Sons, Inc.

King James Bible. (1976). Thomas Nelson, Inc. (original work published 1798).

AskDoctorPam – About Mental Health

www.ingramcontent.com/pod-product-compliance
Lightning Source LLC
Chambersburg PA
CBHW031534210526
45464CB00013B/609